Contents

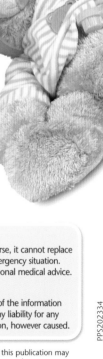

Edition 4.0

IMPORTANT
This book is designed as a learning guide to a full first aid course, it cannot replace 'hands on' training in the vital skills of dealing with an emergency situation. If you suspect illness or injury, you should always seek professional medical advice.

DISCLAIMER
Whilst every effort has been made to ensure the accuracy of the information contained within this book, the author does not accept any liability for any inaccuracies or for any subsequent mistreatment of any person, however caused.

© 2007. First on Scene Training Ltd. All Rights Reserved. No part of this publication may be reproduced, stored in a retrieval system, or transmitted in any form or by any means, electronic, mechanical, photocopying, recording or otherwise, without the prior written permission of the copyright owner. Tel. 0845 644 3305. www.FirstAidMadeEasy.co.uk

PPS202334

D0257755

Emergency action plan

Planning for an emergency

The prevention of accidents is obviously preferable to giving first aid. Nothing can replace adequate supervision of a child in a friendly and relaxed environment. Now and again however, accidents and illness do happen, and you may be called upon to give first aid to a child in your care.

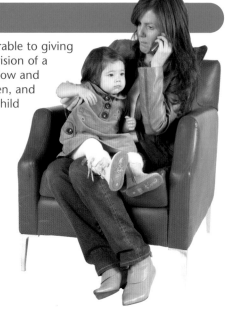

It is important, therefore, to make a plan for how you would deal with such an emergency situation:

- What would you do if a child in your care has a serious accident or sudden illness?
- What if that accident or illness happened to you?

Take some time to consider what your actions would be if an emergency happened whilst you were caring for children:

Useful things to consider when you make your plan:

- Access to a telephone *(and a back up if it's out of order)*.
- Do you have someone who can care for the children if you have to leave them?
- Do you have a fully equipped first aid box that is easy for you and others to find?
- Are the children's record forms to hand so you can take them to hospital with you?
- Do you have a fire escape plan? What if the exits or stairs were blocked? Do you have an agreed 'meeting' point outside?
- Do the parents know what to expect if there is an emergency and what you will ask of them?
- Make a list of important phone numbers that you and others can find easily:
  - Parents of the children *(home, work and mobile)*.
  - Doctors surgery *(yours and the children's)*.
  - NHS Direct advice line *(0845 4647)*.
  - Emergency back up person.
  - Ofsted advisor or Childminding Network Co-ordinator.
- Have you been on a first aid course to learn what to do in an emergency? *(Just reading this book is not enough!)*.

Priorities of treating a patient

When dealing with a child who is injured or ill it is important to treat the most serious conditions first.

All animal life needs a constant supply of oxygen to survive. If that oxygen is taken away for any reason, brain cells will start to die within 3 to 4 minutes.

The priorities of treatment are therefore aimed firstly at getting oxygen into the blood stream, ensuring that the blood is circulating around the body, and then preventing the loss of that blood.

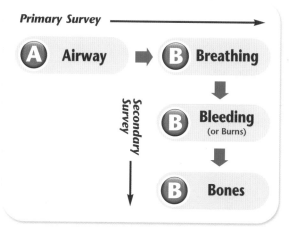

Primary Survey

(A) Airway ➡ **(B) Breathing**

Secondary Survey

(B) Bleeding (or Burns)

(B) Bones

The first priority with any patient is to make sure the **Airway** is open and then to check they are **Breathing** normally *(A and B)*. If the patient is breathing normally, this means that their heart must also be beating, so blood is being circulated around the body. As the **A** and **B** check is carried out first, we call it the *'primary survey'*.

Once you are happy that the casualty is **Breathing** normally and oxygen is being circulated around the body, the next priority is to deal with any major **Bleeding** because you need to maintain enough blood to circulate the oxygen around. After these steps, the next priority is to deal with any broken **Bones** *(BBB)*. The check for bleeding and then broken bones is called the *'secondary survey'*.

Multiple casualties

*The **BBB** rule can be used for multiple casualties, to decide who needs treatment first. A rough 'rule of thumb' is that the casualty who is the quietest needs treatment first, whereas the one making the most noise (trying to get your attention) is the least serious!*

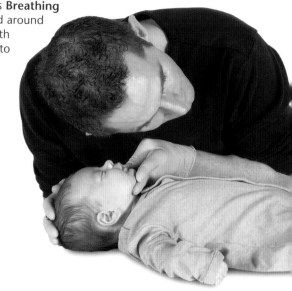

Emergency action plan

It is important to have an action plan for emergencies. This flow chart guides you through the actions to be taken when dealing with a patient. All the topics, such as the 'recovery position' and 'resuscitation' are covered later in the book.

 DANGER?
Look for any further danger.

YES → **Remove Danger**
Make the scene safe.
Do not take risks.

NO

 Response?
Shout and gently shake or tap the casualty.

YES → **History**
Find out what has happened.

↓

Signs and Symptoms
How does the patient feel or look?
Try to work out what's wrong.

↓

Treatment
Remember – if you're not sure, always seek professional medical advice.

NO

Help!
Shout for help but don't leave the casualty yet.

 Airway
Open the airway by tilting the head back and lifting the chin.

 Normal Breathing?
Look, listen and feel for no more than 10 seconds.

YES → **Secondary Survey**
Check for bleeding, injuries and clues *(page 14)*.

↓

Recovery Position
• Recovery Position *(page 15)*.
• **Dial 999 if not already done.**
• Monitor Airway and Breathing.
• Keep the casualty warm.

NO

Dial 999
(If the patient is a child or baby and you are on your own, resuscitate for 1 minute first).

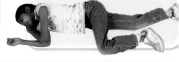

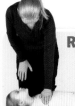 **Resuscitation**

30 to 2 ←→

• For a child or baby – give 5 initial rescue breaths.
• Give 30 chest compressions, then 2 rescue breaths.
• Continue giving cycles of 30 compressions to 2 rescue breaths.
• Only stop to recheck the patient if they start breathing **normally** – otherwise do not interrupt resuscitation.
• If there is more than one rescuer, change over every 2 minutes.

Resuscitation foreword

Recent studies have found that many children do not receive resuscitation because potential rescuers fear causing them harm. This fear was increased in some cases because the rescuer knew that the guidelines for child resuscitation were different from adults.

It is, of course, far better to perform the 'adult sequence' of resuscitation on a child who is unresponsive and not breathing than to do nothing at all.

Studies have also shown that the more 'steps' in the resuscitation sequence a first aider has to learn, the less likely they will be able to recall them in a 'real' cardiac arrest situation.

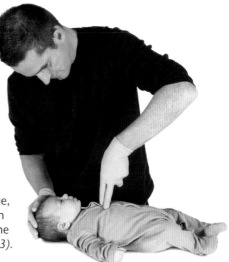

For these reasons, the latest resuscitation guidelines focus on minimising the number of steps to be learned and first aiders can now use the 'adult sequence' of resuscitation on a child or baby who is unresponsive and not breathing. There are, however, minor modifications to the sequence that can make it even more suitable for use with children.

The adult sequence is given in detail over the page, then the minor modifications that can make it even more suitable for children have been included in the child and baby resuscitation section *(pages 10 to 13)*.

Minor modifications for children:

As soon as you identify that the child is 'unresponsive' and 'not breathing normally':

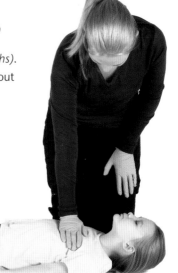

- Give **five** initial 'rescue breaths' *(described on page 8)* before starting chest compressions *(then continue resuscitation at the ratio of **30** compressions to **2** breaths)*.
- **If you are on your own** – perform resuscitation for about 1 minute before going for help.
- When performing 'chest compressions' *(described on page 7)*, compress the chest by about one-third of its depth:
  - For a baby under 1 year, use **two fingers**.
  - For a child over 1 year, use **one or two hands** as required to depress the chest a third of its depth.

Resuscitation – (Cardio Pulmonary Resuscitation)

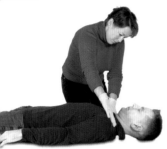

Gently shake the shoulders and shout.

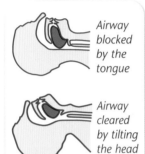

Airway blocked by the tongue

Airway cleared by tilting the head

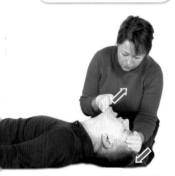

Tilt the head back and lift the chin to open the airway.

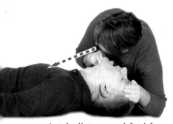

Look, listen and feel for normal breathing.

Resuscitation

 ### Danger – *make sure it's safe to help*

- Check that it is safe for you to help the casualty. Do not put yourself at risk in any way.
- If possible remove any danger from the casualty, or if not, can you safely move the casualty from the danger?
- Find out what's happened – and make sure you are still safe.
- Check how many casualties there are. Can you cope?

 ### Response – *are they conscious?*

- Gently shake the shoulders and ask loudly 'are you alright?'
- If there is no response, shout for help immediately, but do not leave the casualty yet.

 ### Airway – *open the airway*

Carefully open the airway by using 'head tilt' and 'chin lift':

- Place your hand on the forehead and gently tilt the head back.
- With your fingertips under the point of the casualty's chin, lift the chin to open the airway *(see diagram)*.

 ### Breathing – *check for normal breathing*

Keeping the airway open, check to see if the breathing is normal. Take no more than 10 seconds to do this:

- **Look** at the chest and abdomen for movement.
- **Listen** for the sounds of breathing *(more than the occasional gasp)*.
- **Feel** for breath on your cheek or movement of the chest or abdomen.

If the casualty **is** breathing **normally**, carry out a secondary survey and place them in the recovery position *(pages 14 and 15)*.

NOTE: *In the first few minutes after cardiac arrest, a casualty may be barely breathing, or taking infrequent, noisy gasps. Do not confuse this with normal breathing. If you have any doubt whether breathing is normal, act as if it is **not** normal.*

If the casualty is not breathing normally:

Ask someone to **dial 999 for an ambulance** or, if you are on your own, do this yourself; you may need to leave the casualty.

Start chest compressions as follows:

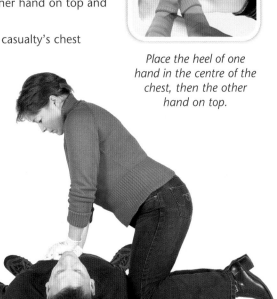

* Place the heel of one hand in the centre of the casualty's chest, then place the heel of your other hand on top and interlock your fingers *(see diagram).*

* Position yourself vertically above the casualty's chest with your arms straight.

Place the heel of one hand in the centre of the chest, then the other hand on top.

* Press down on the breastbone 4 to 5cm *(1¹/₂ to 2 inches)* then release the pressure without losing contact between your hands and the chest *(chest compression)*. Ensure that pressure is not applied over the casualty's ribs. Don't apply pressure over the upper abdomen or the bottom end of the breastbone.

* Compression and release should take an equal amount of time.

* **Do 30 chest compressions** at a rate of 100 per minute.

* **Now combine chest compressions with rescue breaths** *(over the page).*

Arms straight and shoulders above your hands. Depress the chest 4 to 5cm.

Now combine chest compressions with rescue breaths – *over the page*

NOTE: *Ideally the casualty needs to be on a firm flat surface to perform chest compressions (not a bed). One way to remove someone from a low bed is to unhook the bed sheets and use them to slide the casualty carefully to the floor. Get help if you can and be very careful not to injure yourself or the casualty. Do not move the casualty if you do not think it's safe to do so – remove the pillows and attempt CPR on the bed instead.*

Resuscitation – (CPR)

Combine chest compressions with rescue breaths:

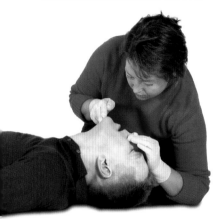

Nip the nose.

- Open the airway again, using head tilt and chin lift.
- Nip the soft part of the casualty's nose closed. Allow the mouth to open, but maintain chin lift.
- Take a normal breath and seal your lips around the casualty's mouth.
- Blow steadily into the casualty's mouth, whilst watching for the chest to rise *(rescue breath)*. Take about one second to make the chest rise.
- Keeping the airway open, remove your mouth. Take a breath of fresh air and watch for the casualty's chest to fall as air comes out.
- Re-seal your mouth and give another rescue breath *(two in total)*.
- Return your hands without delay to the correct position on the breastbone and give another 30 chest compressions *(then 2 more rescue breaths)*.
- **Continue repeating cycles of 30 chest compressions and 2 rescue breaths.**
- Only stop to recheck the casualty if they start breathing normally – otherwise don't interrupt resuscitation.

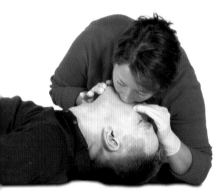

Rescue breaths.

If there is more than one rescuer, change over every two minutes to prevent fatigue. Ensure the minimum of delay as you change over.

If your rescue breaths don't make the chest rise effectively:

Give another 30 chest compressions, then before your next attempt:

- Check the casualty's mouth and remove any visible obstruction.
- Recheck that there is adequate head tilt and chin lift.
- Do not attempt more than 2 breaths each time before returning to chest compressions.

Continue resuscitation until:

- Qualified help arrives to takes over,
- The casualty starts breathing normally, or
- You become exhausted.

Chest compression only resuscitation

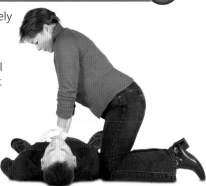

When an **adult** casualty suffers a cardiac arrest, it is likely that there is residual oxygen left in the blood stream.

If you are unable *(or unwilling)* to give rescue breaths, give 'chest compressions only' resuscitation, as this will circulate any residual oxygen in the blood stream, so it is better than no resuscitation at all.

- If chest compressions only are given, these should be continuous at a rate of 100 per minute.
- Stop to recheck the casualty only if they start breathing normally – otherwise do not interrupt resuscitation.
- If there is more than one rescuer, change over every two minutes to prevent fatigue. Ensure the minimum of delay as you change over.

Vomiting

It is common for a patient who has stopped breathing to vomit whilst they are collapsed. This is a passive action in the unconscious person, so you may not hear or see it happening. You might not find out until you give a rescue breath *(as the air comes back out of the patient it makes gurgling noises).*

- If the patient has vomited, turn them onto their side, tip the head back and allow the vomit to run out.
- Clean the face of the patient then continue resuscitation, using a protective face barrier if possible.

Hygiene during resuscitation:

- Wipe the lips clean.
- If possible use a protective barrier such as a 'resusci–aid'. *(This is particularly important if the patient suffers from any serious infectious disease such as TB or S.A.R.S.).*
- As a last resort some plastic with a hole in it, or a handkerchief, may help to prevent direct contact.
- If you are still in doubt about the safety of performing rescue breaths, give 'chest compression only' resuscitation *(see above).*
- Wear protective gloves if available and wash your hands afterwards.

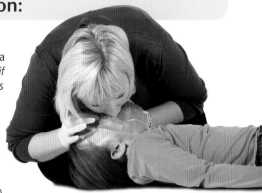

Using a protective barrier.

Resuscitation – Child (over 1 year)

NOTE: *The minor modifications to the adult sequence of resuscitation (page 5) that can make it even more suitable for children have been included below.*

REMEMBER: *If you are unsure, it is better to perform the adult sequence of resuscitation on a child (who is unresponsive and not breathing) than to do nothing at all.*

Child resuscitation

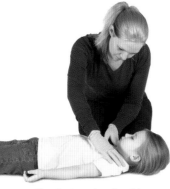

D Danger

- Check that it is safe for you to help. Do not put yourself at risk.

R Response

- Gently tap the shoulders and shout 'are you alright?'
- If there is no response, shout for help, but don't leave the child just yet.

Gently tap the shoulders and shout.

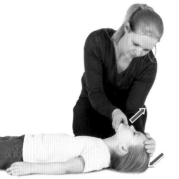

A Airway

Carefully open the airway by using 'head tilt' and 'chin lift':

- Place your hand on the forehead and gently tilt the head back.
- With your fingertips under the point of the chin, lift the chin to open the airway.

B Breathing

Keeping the airway open, look, listen and feel to see if the breathing is normal. Take no more than 10 seconds to do this.

- If the child is breathing **normally**, carry out a secondary survey and place them in the recovery position *(pages 14 and 15)*.

Open the airway.

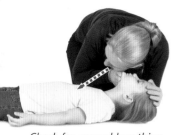

Check for normal breathing.

If the child is not breathing normally:

- Ask someone to **dial 999 for an ambulance** immediately, but if you are on your own, and you have to leave the child to dial 999, carry out resuscitation for about 1 minute first:
- Keep the airway open by tilting the head and lifting the chin.
- Nip the nose and seal your mouth around the child's mouth.
- Give 5 initial rescue breaths *(blow in just enough air to make the child's chest visibly rise).*

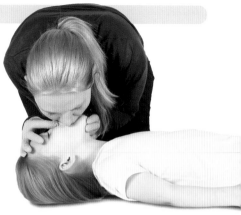

Rescue breaths.

Combine rescue breaths with chest compressions:

- Use 1 or 2 hands as required to depress the chest a third of its depth.
- Give 30 chest compressions at a rate of 100 per minute.
- Open the airway again by tilting the head and lifting the chin, then give 2 more rescue breaths.
- **Continue repeating cycles of 30 compressions to 2 rescue breaths.**
- Only stop to recheck the child if they start breathing normally – otherwise do not interrupt resuscitation.

If your rescue breaths don't make the chest rise effectively:

Give another 30 chest compressions, then before your next attempt:

- Check inside the mouth and remove any visible obstruction *(but don't reach blindly into the back of the throat).*
- Recheck there is adequate head tilt and chin lift.
- Do not attempt more than 2 breaths each time before returning to chest compressions.

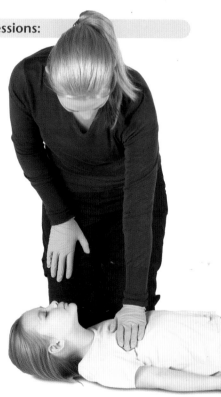

Use 1 or 2 hands to depress the chest by one third of its depth.

NOTE: *If there is more than one rescuer, change over every two minutes to prevent fatigue. Ensure the minimum of delay as you change over.*

Resuscitation – Baby (under 1 year)

NOTE: *The minor modifications to the adult sequence of resuscitation (page 5) that can make it even more suitable for children and babies have been included below.*

REMEMBER: *If you are unsure, it is better to perform the adult sequence of resuscitation on a baby (who is unresponsive and not breathing) than to do nothing at all.*

Baby resuscitation

D Danger

- Check that it is safe for you to help. Do not put yourself at risk.

R Response

- Gently tap the shoulders and shout to try and wake the baby.
- If there is no response, shout for help, but don't leave the baby just yet.

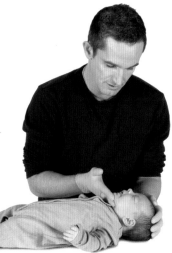

Open the airway.

A Airway

Carefully open the airway by using 'head tilt' and 'chin lift':

- Place your hand on the forehead and gently tilt the head back. Do not over-extend the neck.
- With your fingertips under the point of the chin, gently lift the chin to open the airway.

B Breathing

Keeping the airway open, look, listen and feel to see if the breathing is normal. Take no more than 10 seconds to do this.

- If the baby is breathing **normally**, consider injuries and place them in the recovery position *(page 15)*.

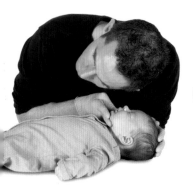

Check for normal breathing.

If the baby is not breathing normally:

- Ask someone to **dial 999 for an ambulance** immediately, but if you are on your own, and you have to leave the baby to dial 999, carry out resuscitation for about 1 minute first:
- Keep the airway open by tilting the head and lifting the chin *(do not over-extend the neck)*.
- Seal your mouth around the baby's mouth and nose.
- Give 5 initial rescue breaths *(blow in just enough air to make the chest visibly rise)*. **Take care not to over inflate the lungs**.

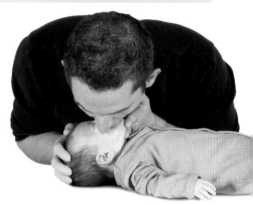

Rescue breaths.

Combine rescue breaths with chest compressions:

- Use 2 fingers to depress the chest a third of its depth.
- Give 30 chest compressions at a rate of 100 per minute.
- Open the airway again by tilting the head and lifting the chin, then give 2 more rescue breaths.
- **Continue repeating cycles of 30 compressions to 2 rescue breaths.**
- Only stop to recheck the child if they start breathing normally – otherwise don't interrupt resuscitation.

If your rescue breaths don't make the chest rise effectively:

Give another 30 chest compressions, then before your next attempt:

- Check inside the mouth and remove any visible obstruction *(but don't reach blindly into the back of the throat)*.
- Recheck there is adequate head tilt and chin lift.
- Do not attempt more than 2 breaths each time before returning to chest compressions.

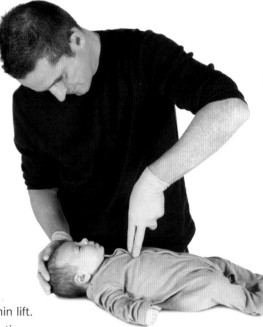

Use 2 fingers to depress the chest by one third of its depth.

Unconsciousness – checking a patient

The Primary and Secondary Survey methods of checking a patient give us a systematic order in which to deal with the most urgent problems first, then move on to find other clues.

Primary survey

When you check for **D**anger, **R**esponse, **A**irway and **B**reathing this is called the 'Primary Survey' *(see page 6)*.

The primary survey ensures that the patient is breathing, so it should be carried out first.

Once you are sure that the patient is breathing effectively, it is safe to move on and carry out a secondary survey:

Secondary survey

Check first for major bleeding and then for broken bones. The check should be done quickly and systematically.

If you are concerned about the airway for any reason *(e.g. vomiting)*, put the patient in the recovery position immediately *(opposite)*.

Bleeding	Do a quick head to toe check for bleeding. Control any major bleeding that you find *(page 23)*.
Head and neck	Clues to injury could be bruising, swelling, deformity, or bleeding. Check the whole head and face. Feel the back of the neck. Has the patient had an accident that might have injured the neck? *(page 36)*.
Shoulders and chest	Place your hands on opposite shoulders and compare them. Run your fingers down the collar bones checking for signs of a fracture *(page 32)*. Gently squeeze and rock the ribs.
Abdomen and pelvis	Push the abdomen with the palm of your hand to check for abnormality or response to pain. Gently check the pelvis for signs of a fracture. Look for incontinence or bleeding.
Legs and arms	Check each leg, then each arm, for signs of a fracture. Look for other clues *(medic alert bracelets, needle marks etc)*.
Pockets	Look for clues and make sure nothing will injure the patient as you roll them into the recovery position. *(Have a witness if you remove items from pockets and be very careful if you suspect there could be sharp objects such as needles)*. Loosen any tight clothing.
Recovery	Place the patient in the recovery position *(opposite)*. Be careful not to cause further damage to any suspected injuries.

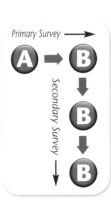

Primary Survey ⟶

Ⓐ ➡ Ⓑ

Secondary Survey

Ⓑ

Ⓑ

Ⓑ

Remember the priorities of treatment? (page 3)

The recovery position

Before you move a patient, it is important to consider the 'mechanics of injury'. Try to work out what happened and what injuries this could have caused.

- If you suspect neck injury, get someone to help you keep the head in line with the body at all times *(see page 36)*.
- If you have to use the recovery position, try not to move any suspected injuries.

When an unconscious person is lying on their back, there are 2 main dangers that can compromise the airway:

> The Tongue: Touching the back of the throat.
>
> Vomit: If the patient is sick.

By placing the casualty in the recovery position, the tongue will not fall backwards, so it won't block the airway. If the casualty is sick, the vomit will run out of the mouth and keep the airway clear.

To place someone in the recovery position:

- Remove the patient's glasses.
- Kneel beside the patient and make sure that both their legs are straight.
- Place the arm nearest you out at right angles to the body, elbow bent with palm uppermost *(picture 1)*.
- Bring the patient's far arm across their chest, and hold the back of that hand against their cheek *(picture 2)*.
- With your other hand, grasp the far leg just above the knee, and pull it up, keeping their foot on the ground *(picture 3)*.
- Keeping their hand pressed against their cheek, pull on the leg to roll them towards you, onto their side.
- Adjust the upper leg so that both the hip and the knee are bent at right angles *(picture 4)*.
- Tilt the head back to make sure the airway remains open.
- Call for an ambulance if this has not already been done.
- Check breathing regularly. If breathing stops, turn the patient onto their back again and perform resuscitation.

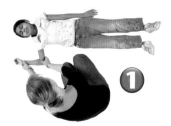

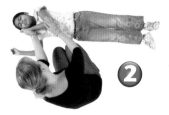

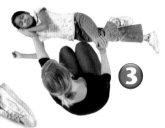

Airway and breathing problems

Choking – CHILD *(over 1 year)*

Firstly encourage the child to cough. If the choking is only mild, this will clear the obstruction and the child should be able to speak to you.

If the obstruction is not cleared:

1 Back slaps

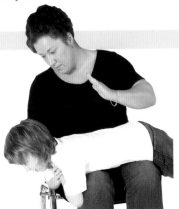

- **Shout for help**, but don't leave the child yet.
- Lean the child over your knee or bend them forwards, so the head is lower than the chest.
- Give up to 5 firm blows between the shoulder blades with the palm of your hand. Check between blows and stop if you clear the obstruction.

If the obstruction is still not cleared:

2 Abdominal thrusts

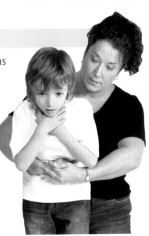

- Kneel or stand behind the child. Place both your arms around their waist.
- Make a fist with one hand, and place it just above the belly button *(below the ribs)* with your thumb inwards. Grasp this fist with your other hand.
- Thrust sharply inwards and upwards. Try this up to 5 times. Check between thrusts and stop if you clear the obstruction.

If the obstruction is still not cleared:

3 Repeat steps 1 and 2

- Keep repeating steps 1 and 2.
- If the treatment seems ineffective, shout for help. Ask someone to **dial 999 for an ambulance**, but don't interrupt the treatment yet.

If the child becomes unconscious:

NOTE: *information on when to refer the patient to a doctor is on page 18.*

- Place the child on a firm, flat surface.
- **START CPR** – follow the sequence on page 11 after the heading 'if the child is not breathing normally'.

Choking – BABY *(under 1 year)*

The baby may attempt to cough. If the choking is only mild, this will clear the obstruction – the baby may cry and should now be able to breathe effectively.

If the obstruction is not cleared:

1 Back slaps

- **Shout for help**, but don't leave the baby yet.
- Lay the baby over your arm, face down, legs either side of your elbow with the head below the chest *(see picture)*.
- Give up to 5 blows between the shoulder blades with the palms of your fingers. Check between blows and stop if you clear the obstruction.

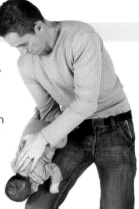

If the obstruction is still not cleared:

2 Chest thrusts

- Turn the baby over, chest uppermost, *(by laying them on your other arm)* and lower the head below the level of the chest.
- Using two fingers on the chest, give up to 5 chest thrusts. These are similar to chest compressions, but sharper in nature and delivered at a slower rate. Check between thrusts and stop if you clear the obstruction.

NEVER *perform abdominal thrusts on a baby.*

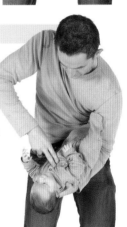

If the obstruction is still not cleared:

3 Repeat steps 1 and 2

- Keep repeating steps 1 and 2.
- If the treatment seems ineffective, shout for help. Ask someone to **dial 999 for an ambulance**, but don't interrupt the treatment yet.

If the baby becomes unconscious:

- Place the baby on a firm, flat surface.
- **START CPR** – follow the sequence on page 13 after the heading 'if the baby is not breathing normally'.

NOTE: information on when to refer the patient to a doctor is on page 18.

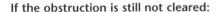

Airway and breathing problems

Choking – ADULT

Firstly, encourage the patient to cough. If the choking is only mild, this will clear the obstruction and the patient should be able to speak to you.

If the obstruction is not cleared:

1 Back slaps

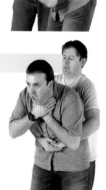

- **Shout for help**, but don't leave the patient yet.
- Bend the casualty over so the head is lower than the chest.
- Give up to 5 firm blows between the shoulder blades with the palm of your hand. Check between blows and stop if you clear the obstruction.

If the obstruction is still not cleared:

2 Abdominal thrusts

- Stand behind the casualty. Place both your arms around their waist.
- Make a fist with one hand and place it over the abdomen *(below the ribs)* with your thumb inwards.
- Grasp this fist with your other hand, then pull sharply inwards and upwards. Do this up to 5 times. Check between thrusts and stop if you clear the obstruction.

If the obstruction is still not cleared:

3 Repeat steps 1 and 2

- Repeat steps 1 and 2.
- If the treatment seems ineffective, shout for help. Ask someone to **dial 999 for an ambulance**, but don't interrupt the treatment whilst the patient is still conscious.

If the patient becomes unconscious:

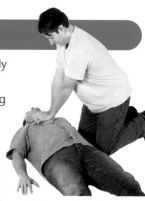

- Support the casualty carefully to the ground and immediately **dial 999 for an ambulance** *(if not already done)*.
- **Start CPR** – follow the sequence on page 7 after the heading 'if the casualty is not breathing normally:'

Abdominal thrusts can cause serious internal injuries, so send the patient to see a doctor.
After successful treatment, patients with a persistent cough, difficulty swallowing or with the feeling of an 'object still stuck in the throat' should also see a doctor.

If the patient becomes unconscious – start CPR.

Allergic reaction (anaphylaxis)

Anaphylaxis is an extremely dangerous allergic reaction. The name 'anaphylaxis' means '*without protection*'. The condition is caused by a massive over-reaction of the body's immune system.

Severe anaphylactic reactions are very rare, but if the airway or breathing are affected, death can occur in minutes.

Common allergies are to things such as peanuts, egg or milk products, insect stings, seafoods or drugs *(such as penicillin)*.

The main chemical that the immune cells release if they detect a 'foreign protein' is called '**histamine**'. It is the massive quantities of histamine being released in the body during an anaphylactic reaction that cause the signs and symptoms of the condition:

Signs and symptoms

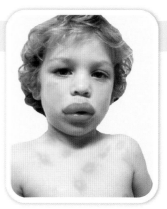

- Swelling of the face, tongue, lips, neck and eyes.
- Difficulty breathing *(the child may have the equivalent of an asthma attack as well as a swollen airway)*.
- Fast, weak pulse.
- Red, blotchy rash on the skin.
- Anxiety.

Treatment of anaphylaxis

- **Dial 999 for an ambulance**. Pass on as much information as you can about the condition of the patient.
- Help the conscious child to sit up to help their breathing.
- Monitor the child's breathing until the ambulance arrives.
- If the child becomes unconscious – check **Airway** and **Breathing**. Resuscitate as necessary *(pages 10 to 13)*.
- A child who has suffered a previous anaphylactic reaction may carry a syringe of adrenaline *(Epi-Pen)*. This can save the child's life if it's given promptly. If the child is not old enough to administer this on their own, an adult should receive training from a qualified Nurse or Doctor, to enable them to administer the medication.

Picture: many thanks to the Anaphylaxis Campaign.
www.anaphylaxis.org.uk   © MedicalMediaKits.com

Asthma

Asthma is a condition caused by an allergic reaction in the lungs, often to substances such as dust, traffic fumes or animal hair.

Muscles surrounding the tiny wind pipes in the lungs go into spasm and constrict, making it very difficult for the child to breathe.

Most asthma patients carry medication around with them, usually in the form of an inhaler. Ask the child's parents, but usually the *blue* inhaler is for 'emergency' use, opening the wind pipes to relieve the condition.

An asthma attack is a traumatic experience for any child, so reassurance and a calm approach from the first aider is essential.

Possible signs and symptoms

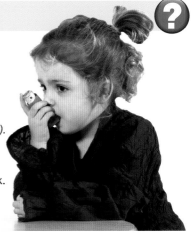

- Difficulty breathing.
- Wheezy breath sounds, originating from the lungs.
- Difficulty speaking (*will need to take a breath in the middle of a sentence*).
- Pale, clammy skin.
- Grey or blue lips and skin (*if the attack is very severe*).
- Use of muscles in the neck and upper chest to help the child breathe.
- The child may become exhausted in a severe attack.
- The child may become unconscious and stop breathing in a prolonged attack.

Treatment of asthma attack

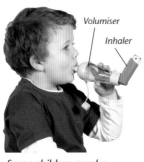

Volumiser

Inhaler

Some children need a 'volumiser' because they can't take their inhaler all in one breath.

- Keep calm and be reassuring towards the child.
- Help the child to sit upright, leaning on a table or chair if necessary.
- Help the child to take their own medication.
- Try to take the child's mind off the attack – make conversation.
- If the attack is prolonged, the attack appears to be very severe, or the medication is not effective, **dial 999 for an ambulance.**
- Cold winter air can make an attack worse, so don't take them outside for fresh air!
- Keep the child upright – even if they become too weak to sit up on their own. Only lay an asthma attack patient down if they become deeply unconscious.

Croup

Croup is a condition usually suffered by young children, where the voice box and wind pipe become infected and swollen. The attacks, which often occur during the night, can appear very alarming, but nearly always clear without causing the child any lasting harm.

Possible signs and symptoms

- Difficult distressed breathing.
- A loud pitched, or whistling noise as the child breathes.
- A short 'barking' type cough.
- Pale, clammy skin, possibly blue tinges to the lips.
- Use of muscles in the neck and upper chest to help the child breathe.

Treatment of croup

- Keep calm – panic will distress the child and make the attack worse.
- Sit the child up and reassure them.
- Create a steamy atmosphere in the room – boil a kettle, run a hot bath or shower. Beware, hot water and steam can burn!
- If the condition eases, keep the room where the child rests humid. This may prevent a further attack. Stay with the child all night.
- Call the doctor. If the attack is severe, does not ease, the child has blue tinged lips or a temperature, **dial 999 for an ambulance.**

NEVER put your fingers down the throat of a child that appears to be suffering from croup. There is a small chance that the condition could be 'epiglottitis'. If this is the case, the epiglottis may swell even more, totally blocking the airway.

Drowning

A child who drowns does not usually breathe in large amounts of water. The child will usually swallow large amounts of water, which might then be vomited as they are rescued or resuscitation takes place.

Other factors may contribute to the cause of drowning, for example hypothermia, or an underlying medical condition such as epilepsy.

Treatment of drowning

- Do not put yourself at risk. **'Reach or throw – don't GO'.**
- If possible keep the child horizontal during rescue.
- Check **Airway** and **Breathing**. Resuscitate if necessary.
- **Dial 999 for an ambulance.**

ALWAYS dial 999 for an ambulance, even if the child appears to recover. Just a tiny amount of water in the lungs can cause a delayed reaction of sudden, severe difficulty breathing. This is called 'secondary drowning'.

Wounds and bleeding

How much blood do we have?

The amount of blood in our body varies in relation to our size, so a child or baby will have much less blood than an adult.

A rough rule of thumb is that a person has approximately one pint of blood per stone in body weight *(but the rule doesn't work for someone who is overweight)*.

How much blood loss is critical?

The body can compensate if it is losing blood. It does this by:

- Closing down the blood supply to non-emergency areas of the body *(including the skin and digestive system)*.
- Speeding up the heart to maintain blood pressure.

Blood vessels can only close down so much, and the heart can only go so fast, so there is a limit to the amount of blood loss the body can compensate for. The body can no longer compensate after **one third** of its blood has been lost. After this amount, the blood pressure falls quickly, the blood supply to the brain fails, and death will result.

Particular care is needed for a child who has lost blood, because one third of their blood supply will be much less than that of an adult. The critical blood loss for a baby weighing one stone for example, is just one third of a pint!

Shock

The definition of shock is *'a lack of oxygen to the tissues of the body, which is caused by a fall in blood volume or blood pressure'*.

Severe bleeding can result in shock, which can kill. If the child has lost a large quantity of blood this can cause a reduction in blood supply to the brain *(don't forget that children can't afford to lose as much blood as adults!)*.

Some signs of shock are:

- Pale clammy skin *(with blue or grey tinges if it's severe)*.
- Dizziness or passing out *(especially if they try to stand or sit up)*.
- A fast, weak pulse.
- Rapid shallow breathing.

If a large amount of blood has been lost, you can help the flow of blood to the brain by laying the child down and raising their legs in the air. Keep the child warm, give nothing by mouth and **dial 999 for an ambulance.**

Internal bleeding

Internal bleeding is a serious condition, yet it can be very difficult to recognise in its early stages. Severe internal bleeding can result from injuries to the upper leg, pelvis, abdomen or a lung.

Suspect internal bleeding after an accident if the signs of shock develop *(opposite)*, yet there is no other obvious cause *(such as external bleeding)*.

- **Dial 999 for an ambulance and treat the child for shock as necessary.**

Treatment of bleeding

The aims of treatment for bleeding are firstly to stop the bleeding, preventing the child from going into shock *(opposite)*, and then to prevent infection.

'S.E.E.P.' will help you to remember the steps of treatment:

Sit or lay
Sit or lay the child down. Place them in a position that is appropriate to the location of the wound and the extent of their bleeding.

Examine
Examine the wound. Look for foreign objects, and note how the wound is bleeding. Remember what it looks like, so you can describe it to medical staff when it's covered with a bandage.

Elevate
Elevate the wound. Ensure that the wound is above the level of the heart, using gravity to reduce the blood flow to the injury.

Pressure
Apply direct pressure over the wound to stem the bleeding. If there is an embedded object in the wound, you may be able to apply pressure at either side of the object.

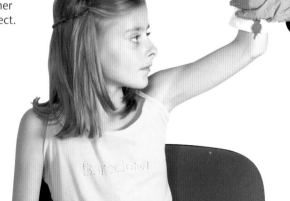

ALWAYS *wear protective gloves when dealing with wounds and bleeding!*

Wounds and bleeding

Dressings

A dressing should be sterile and just large enough to cover the wound. It should be absorbent and preferably made of material which won't stick to the clotting blood *(a 'low-adherent' dressing)*.

A firmly applied dressing is sufficient to stem bleeding from the majority of wounds, but the dressing should not restrict blood flow to the rest of the limb *(check the circulation at the far side of the dressing)*.

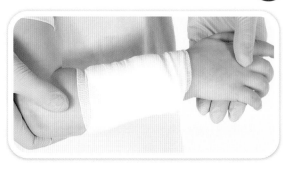

Extra pressure 'by hand' and elevation may be necessary for severe bleeding. If the dressing becomes saturated with blood, keep it in place and put another larger dressing on top. If this doesn't work take the dressings off and start again.

For a hand or arm wound it is a good idea to place the arm in an elevated sling after you have dressed it *(page 33)*. This helps with elevating the wound, but also keeps the bandages clean when the child is playing!

NEVER *try to stop bleeding by tying a band around the limb (a tourniquet). It may cause tissue damage or make the bleeding worse.*

NEVER *remove an embedded object – it may be stemming bleeding and further damage may result.*

Amputation

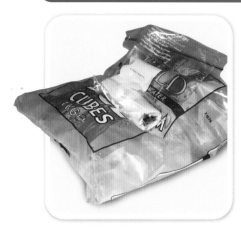

Amputation is the complete or partial severing of a limb, and is extremely traumatic for the casualty. Your priorities are to stop any bleeding, to carefully preserve the amputated body part and to reassure the child.

- Treat the child for bleeding *(page 23)*.
- **Dial 999 for an ambulance.**
- Dress the child's wound with a 'low-adherent', non-fluffy dressing.
- Place the amputated part in a plastic bag, and then put the package on a bag of ice to preserve it. Do not allow the amputated part to come into direct contact with the ice or get wet.

Eye injury

Small particles of dust or dirt can be washed out of a child's eye with cold tap water. Ensure the water runs away from the good eye.

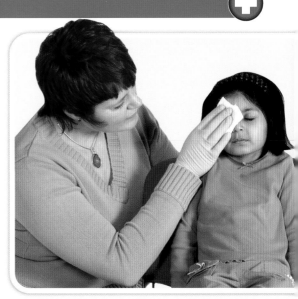

For a more serious eye injury:

- Keep the child still and gently hold a soft sterile dressing over the injured eye. This can be carefully bandaged in place if necessary.

- Tell the child to close their good eye, because any movement of this will cause the injured eye to move also. If necessary bandage the good eye to stop the child using it. Lots of reassurance will be needed!

- Take the child to hospital. **Dial 999 for an ambulance** if necessary.

For chemicals in the eye:

- Wash with copious amounts of clean water, ensuring water runs away from the good eye. **Dial 999 for an ambulance.**

Embedded objects

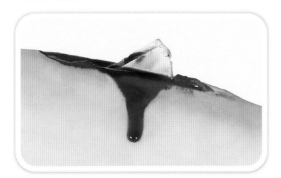

For objects embedded in a wound:

An embedded object in a wound should not be removed because it may be stemming bleeding and further damage may result.

Use sterile dressings and bandages to 'build up' around the protruding object. This will apply pressure around the wound and support the object. Arrange for the child to go to hospital to have the object removed.

For objects embedded in the nose, ear or other orifice:

Do not attempt to remove anything that a child has got stuck in their ear, nose or other orifice. Take the child to hospital where the professionals can remove it safely.

Wounds and bleeding

Other types of wound:

Bruise

Caused by bleeding under the skin. This may be the result of a blunt blow, or bleeding from underlying damage, such as a broken bone.

- Cool the area with an ice pack or running water as soon as possible, for about 10 minutes *(wrap the ice pack in a tea towel or triangular bandage)*.

Graze

The top layers of skin are scraped off, usually as the result of a friction burn or sliding fall. A graze often contains particles of dirt, which could cause infection.

- Wash the graze using clean water and sterile swabs. Do not use cotton wool, antiseptic creams or antiseptic wipes etc. If possible, clean from the centre of the wound outwards, so as not to introduce more dirt into the wound.
- Dress the graze with a sterile low-adherent dressing.

DO NOT use cotton wool, antiseptic creams or antiseptic wipes etc.

Puncture

A stabbing wound. Could be as a result of standing on a nail, or being stabbed. The wound could be very deep and yet appear very small in diameter. Damage may be caused to underlying organs such as the heart or lungs and severe internal bleeding may occur.

- **Dial 999 for an ambulance** if you suspect damage to underlying organs or internal bleeding.
- Never remove an embedded object – it may be stemming bleeding and further damage may result.

NEVER remove an embedded object. It may be stemming bleeding and further damage may result.

Gunshot

Caused by a bullet or other missile, which may be travelling at such speed as to drive into, and then exit the body. A small entry wound could be accompanied by a large 'crater' exit wound. Severe bleeding and damage to organs usually results.

- **Dial 999 for Police and Ambulance.**
- Treat **Airway** and **Breathing** problems first *(pages 10 to 13)*.
- Pack the wound with bulky dressings and try to prevent bleeding. Ideally use wet dressings if they come into contact with internal organs.

Animal bite

Animal bites could be infected with bacteria and
other germs, so it's important to clean the
wound thoroughly to reduce the risk of infection.

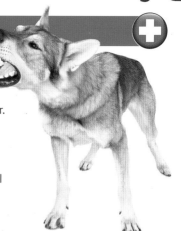

- Clean the wound thoroughly with soap and warm water.
- Treat for bleeding if necessary *(page 23)*.
- Pat the wound dry and cover with a sterile
  low-adherent dressing.
- Seek medical advice. Take or send the child to hospital
  if the wound is large or deep.

Insect sting (bees and wasps)

- Reassure the child. If the sting is visible carefully scrape it off the skin with the blunt
  edge of a knife *(do not use tweezers)*.
- Elevate the injury if possible and apply an ice pack *(wrapped in a tea towel or
  triangular bandage)* for 10 minutes. Seek medical advice if the pain or swelling persist.
- If the sting is in the mouth give an ice cube to suck on, or sips of cold water.
- Keep an eye out for allergic reaction *(see page 19 for more details)*.

Nose bleeds

Weakened or dried out blood vessels in the nose can rupture as a result of a bang
to the nose, picking or blowing it. More serious causes could be high blood pressure
or a fractured skull.

- Sit the child down, head tipped forward.
- Nip the soft part of the nose. Maintain
  constant pressure for 10 minutes.
- Tell the child to breathe through the mouth.
- Give the child a cloth to mop up any blood
  whilst the nose is nipped.
- Advise the child not to breathe through or
  blow their nose for a few hours after the
  bleeding has stopped.
- If bleeding persists, take or send the child
  to hospital in an upright position.
- A child suffering from frequent nose bleeds
  should see the doctor.

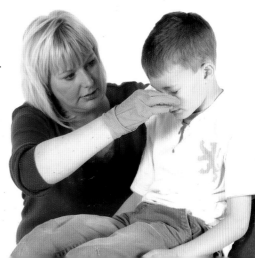

Poisons and burns

Poisoning

A poison can be described as any substance (solid, liquid or gas) that causes damage when it enters the body in sufficient quantity.

A poison can enter the body in 4 ways, it can be:

Ingested	Swallowed.
Inhaled	Breathed in, entering the blood stream very quickly as it passes through the lungs.
Absorbed	Through the skin.
Injected	Through the skin, directly into tissues or a blood vessel.

A poison can either be:

Corrosive	Such as acids, bleach, dishwasher powder, ammonia or petrol.
OR	
Non-corrosive	Such as tablets, drugs, alcohol, plants or perfume.

Treatment

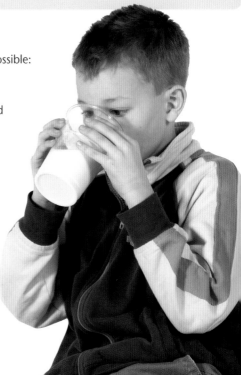

For a corrosive substance:

- Don't endanger yourself – make sure it's safe to help.

- Dilute the substance or wash it away if possible:
  - Substances on the skin – wash away with water *(see burns)*.
  - Swallowed substances – get the child to rinse out their mouth, then give frequent sips of milk or water.

- **Dial 999 for an ambulance.** Give information about the poison if possible. Take advice from the ambulance operator.

- If the child becomes unconscious – open the **Airway** and check for **Breathing**. Resuscitate if necessary using a protective face shield *(page 9)*. If the child is breathing, place them in the recovery position, then dial 999.

NEVER *make the patient vomit.*
This may put the airway in danger.

For a non-corrosive substance:

- **Dial 999 for an ambulance.** Give information about the poison if possible. Take advice from the ambulance operator.

- If the child becomes unconscious – open the **Airway** and check for **Breathing**. Resuscitate if necessary using a protective face shield *(page 9)*. If the child is breathing, place them in the recovery position, then dial 999.

NOTE: *It helps the paramedics if you:*

- *Pass on containers or other information about the substance.*

- *Find out how much has been taken.*

- *Find out when it was taken.*

- *Keep samples of any vomit for hospital analysis.*

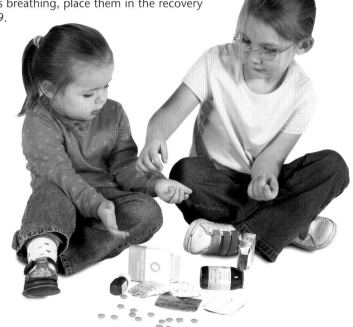

Inhalation of smoke, fumes or other substances:

- Move the child into fresh air if possible.

- Check **Airway** and **Breathing** *(pages 10 to 13)* and resuscitate if necessary.

- If the child is unconscious – place them in the recovery position *(page 15)*.

- **Dial 999 for an ambulance.**

- If the child is conscious and has difficulty breathing, an upright position may help.

- Check for and treat any burns.

- Carefully monitor **Airway** and **Breathing** and resuscitate if necessary.

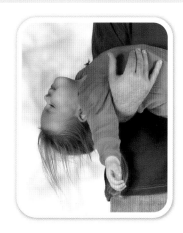

Poisons and burns

Burns or scalds

1 Cool the burn

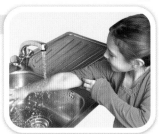

- Cool the burn immediately with cold *(preferably running)* water for 10 minutes.
- If water is not available, any cold harmless liquid *(e.g. milk)* is better than no cooling at all. Do this first then move quickly to a water supply to continue cooling the burn.
- Take care not to cool large areas of burns so much that you induce hypothermia, especially with small children.

2 Remove jewellery and loose clothing

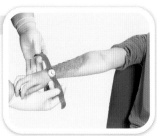

- Remove any constricting items, such as rings and watches, because the area may start to swell.
- Carefully remove loose clothing, taking care that it's not stuck to the burn. *(If the burns are caused by chemicals be careful not to contaminate yourself or other areas of the patient's body).*
- Leave clothing in place if you're not sure that it's loose.

3 Dress the burn

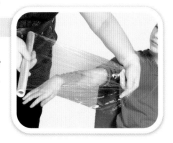

- Dress the burn with a sterile dressing that won't stick to the burn. Cling film is one of the best dressings for a burn – the inside of the roll should be sterile, and it will not stick to the burn *(ensure the wound has been cooled beforehand!).* Do not wrap the burn tightly. Alternatives could be a new, unused plastic bag, or specialised burns dressings.
- It is now recommended that all children with burns are assessed by medical staff, so advise the child's parents to seek medical advice.
- See note *(below right)* on when to seek medical advice.
- If the burn appears severe, or the child has breathed in smoke or fumes, **dial 999 for an ambulance.**

! DO NOT:

- Burst blisters.
- Touch the burn.
- Apply lotions, ointments or fats.
- Apply adhesive tape or dressings.
- Remove clothing that has stuck to the burn.

Seek medical advice if:

- *The burn is larger than 1-inch square.*
- *The patient is a child.*
- *The burn goes all the way around a limb.*
- *Any part of the burn appears to be full thickness.*
- *The burn involves hands, feet, genitals or the face.*
- *You are not sure.*

Electric shock

If a child is electrocuted, an electrical current passes through the body to travel to 'earth'. This can interfere with the body's own electrical impulses, which may cause breathing and even the heart to stop.

You may be able to see a burn where the current entered the body and at the point of exit, but there may be deep internal burns, which are not visible, along the path of the current flow.

An electric shock causes muscles to contract, which might prevent the child from breaking contact with the electricity. In this instance they might still be 'live', so approach with care.

High voltage current

Found in overhead power lines, underground mains cables or railway power lines. Contact with such high voltage electricity is usually fatal, but in any case causes severe burns.

The earth around a faulty high voltage power cable can be live up to 18 metres *(20 yards)* away from the contact point, and the electricity can 'arc' 2 metres *(nearly 7ft)* through the air. Insulating material such as wood or plastic won't protect you.

- Prevent anyone approaching the area *(18 metres)* around the victim.

- **Dial 999 for fire and ambulance** and, if possible, call the emergency number provided by the power company. Do not approach until the power company declare it safe to do so.

- Once it is safe to approach, follow the sequence of resuscitation *(pages 10 to 13)*. If the child is breathing, treat any burns and injuries that you find.

Low voltage current

Caused by contact with domestic voltage electricity, this can still cause serious burns, injuries or even death.

- Ensure the contact with the electricity is broken before you touch the child. Turn off the power at the mains if possible, or unplug the appliance. Do not touch anything metal or that is wet.

- Once you have safely disconnected the power, check **Airway** and **Breathing** *(pages 10 to 13)*.

- If the child is breathing effectively, treat any burns or injuries.

- Take the child to hospital for a check up *(even if they have apparently recovered)*. **Dial 999 for an ambulance** if the child has been unconscious or has electrical burns.

Other serious injuries

Broken bones (?)

Some signs and symptoms of a broken bone are:

Pain At the site of the injury. Other injuries, nerve damage, or pain killers may mask the pain, so beware.

Loss of Power For example not being able to lift anything with a fractured arm.

Unnatural movement This type of fracture is classed as 'unstable' and care should be taken to prevent the bones from moving.

Swelling or bruising Around the site of the injury.

Deformity If a leg is bent in the wrong place, it's broken!

Irregularity Lumps or depressions along the surface of the skin, where the broken ends of the bone overlap.

Crepitus This is the feeling or sound of bone grating on bone if the broken ends rub on each other when the injury is moved about.

Tenderness At the site of the injury.

Treatment of a broken bone ✚

- Keep the injury still and the child warm.
- **Dial 999 for an ambulance if:**
  - There is a suspected injury to the spine, head or neck.
  - The child has difficulty breathing.
  - There is deformity, irregularity or unnatural movement.
  - The bone has come through the skin *(or it looks as if it might do!)*.
  - The child seems to be in a lot of pain.
  - You can't easily get the child to hospital whilst keeping the injury still.
- Don't try bandaging the injury if you have called for an ambulance – just keep it still *(gently cover open wounds with a sterile dressing)*.
- If you can easily get the child to hospital without moving the injury *(and don't need an ambulance)*, gently support the injury and immobilise it if you can.

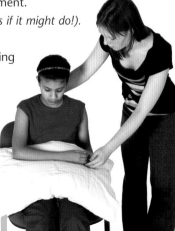

Gently supporting a broken arm.

Sprains and strains

Sprains and strains are injuries to ligaments or muscles. Minor fractures are often mistaken for sprains and strains, so if you're not sure, you should take the child to hospital for an x-ray.

The main aim when treating sprains or strains is to reduce the amount of swelling. This can be done by following '**R.I.C.E.**'

Rest — Rest the injury. Don't allow a child to carry on playing sports.

Ice — Apply an ice pack to the injury as soon as possible. Place a tea towel or triangular bandage between the skin and the ice pack. Do this for 10 minutes, every 2 hours, for 24 hours for maximum effect.

Compression — Apply a firm *(not constrictive)* bandage to the injured area. The bandage can be applied over a crushed ice pack for the first 10 minutes.

Elevation — Elevate the injury.

CAUTION: To prevent frostbite always wrap the ice pack in a cloth and apply it for a maximum of 10 minutes. Allow the skin to return to normal temperature before repeat applications.

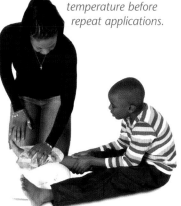

Support sling

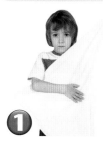
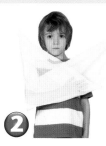
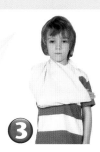

A support sling is often used for supporting lower arm injuries, such as a fractured or sprained wrist.

TIP: Fold a triangular bandage in half for a small child.

Elevated sling

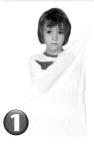
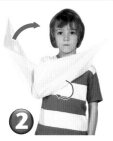
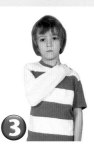

Elevated slings are often used for supporting collar bone and rib injuries. Keep the elbow at the child's side when supporting a collar bone injury.

Other serious injuries

Serious head injuries

Any head injury is potentially a very serious condition. Injuries to the head often lead to unconsciousness, which in turn puts the airway at risk. Permanent damage to the brain may result from a head injury.

Three conditions that may be present with head injuries are 'concussion', 'compression' and 'fractured skull':

Concussion

Concussion is caused by 'shaking' of the brain. The brain is cushioned within the skull by fluid, so if the head receives a blow the brain can bounce from one side to the other, causing widespread disruption to its normal functioning.

- The child may become **unconscious for a short period, after which the levels of consciousness should improve**. The child should recover completely if no complications are present.
- Short term memory loss *(particularly of the accident)* is common.
- Other signs and symptoms include pale, clammy skin and a mild general headache.

Compression

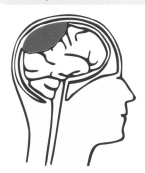

Caused by bleeding or swelling within the skull, compression is a very serious condition, because the brain is placed under extreme pressure *(see diagram)*.

- The child could have a history of recent head injury with apparent recovery, but then deteriorates. **Confusion and levels of consciousness become worse as the condition develops.**
- Other signs and symptoms include flushed, dry skin and intense headache.

Fractured skull

A skull fracture is serious because the broken bone may directly damage the brain, or cause bleeding, which in turn results in compression. Suspect a skull fracture with any child who has received a head injury, especially if they have lowered levels of consciousness.

- **The child may also suffer from concussion or compression, so those signs and symptoms might be present.**
- Other clues include swelling or bruising of the head, around one or both eyes, or behind an ear.

Treatment of serious head injury

REMEMBER: *a blow to the head that is large enough to cause a head injury, can also cause a spinal injury, so treat the child with care! (page 36).*

- **Dial 999 for an ambulance** if the child has been unconscious, their levels of consciousness deteriorate, or you suspect fractured skull.
- Maintain **Airway** and **Breathing** *(pages 10 to 13)*.
- If the child is unconscious, keep them still and constantly monitor their breathing. If you are struggling to keep the airway clear, place them in the recovery position, but keep the head, neck and body in line as you turn the child *(page 36)*.
- If the child is conscious, help them to lie down. Keep the head, neck and body in line in case there is a spinal injury.
- Control any bleeding by applying gentle pressure around the wound, but if there is bleeding or discharge from an ear, don't try to plug the ear or stop the bleeding.
- Look for and treat any other injuries.

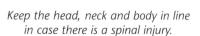

Keep the head, neck and body in line in case there is a spinal injury.

Useful tips for head injury treatment:

- Constantly monitor and record breathing, pulse and the levels of consciousness.
- Even if the child appears to recover, watch out for a subsequent reduction in levels of consciousness *(as this could be the onset of compression)*. Although it's normal for a child to be drowsy after a blow to the head, you should still be able to wake them up.
- Make sure that a concussed child who recovers is not alone for the next 24 hours. Arrange for the child to see a doctor as soon as possible.
- Arrange for the child to go to hospital immediately if they suffer from headache, nausea, vomiting or excessive sleepiness in the next few days.
- Don't allow a concussed child who is playing sports to 'play on' until they have seen a doctor.
- Inform the child's parents, even for the most minor bump to the head. Tell them to look out for the signs of compression and get medical advice if they are worried.

Spinal injury

You should suspect spinal injuries if the child has:

- Sustained a blow to the head, neck or back *(especially resulting in unconsciousness).*
- Fallen from a height *(e.g. a fall from a horse).*
- Dived into shallow water.
- Been in an accident involving speed *(e.g. knocked down or a car accident).*
- Been involved in a 'cave in' accident *(e.g. crushing, or collapsed rugby scrum).*
- Multiple injuries.
- Pain or tenderness in the neck or back after an accident *(beware – pain killers or other severe injuries may mask the pain).*

If you are in any doubt, treat the child as if they have spinal injuries.

Treatment of spinal injury

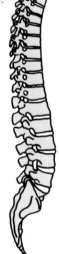

If the child is conscious:

- Reassure the child. Tell them not to move.
- Keep the child in the position you find them. Do not allow them to move, unless they are in severe danger.
- Hold their head still with your hands. Keep the head and neck in line with the upper body *(see picture).*
- **Dial 999 for an ambulance.** Keep the child still and warm until it arrives.

If the child is unconscious:

- If the child is breathing normally this means the airway must be clear, so there is no need to tip the head back, but you will have to gently tip it back and resuscitate if they are not! *(pages 10 to 13).*
- **Dial 999 for an ambulance.**
- Hold the head still with your hands. Keep the head and neck in line with the upper body *(see picture).*
- If you have to **leave** the child *(to dial 999),* if they begin to **vomit,** or if you are concerned 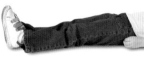 about their **airway** in any way, you should put them into the **recovery position. Keep the head and neck in line with the spine whilst you turn the child.** Get help doing this if you can.
- Keep the child warm and still. Constantly monitor breathing until help arrives. Only move the child if they are in severe danger.

Sickle cell

Sickle cell is a hereditary problem with the red blood cells. A child develops sickle cell disease through genetic information passed on from their parents. If the genetic abnormality is inherited from one parent, it is called the 'sickle cell trait', which is a very mild problem.

If both parents have the sickle cell trait, and pass it on to a child, then the child may develop what is known as 'sickle cell disease', or 'sickle cell anaemia'. This is a more serious condition.

In Britain sickle cell is most common among African and Caribbean people, but it's also found among people originating from the Middle East, India and Pakistan.

The function of red blood cells is mainly to carry oxygen around the body. With sickle cell disease, some of the red blood cells are distorted into a sickle shape, instead of their usual doughnut shape. This distortion disrupts the smooth flow of blood in the narrow blood vessels, leading to blockages. Such a blockage causes an episode known as a 'crisis', which can lead to damage to internal organs. A crisis is also very painful.

Prevention of a crisis can usually be helped by protecting a child from the factors that can induce it. Common triggers are:

- Over-exertion, causing extreme fatigue or tiredness.
- Getting cold, or getting wet.
- Sudden temperature changes *(e.g. from a hot room to cold winter air)*.
- A prolonged infection *(e.g. a chest infection)*.
- Stress or emotional upset.
- Dehydration from not drinking often enough.
- Poor eating habits.

Treatment of sickle cell crisis

You should discuss in advance with the child's parents how to best manage a child with sickle cell, but here are some helpful tips:

- Call the child's parents and arrange for collection.
- Agree measures that can be taken to ease the pain in advance with the child's parents. Get signed consent if medication is required.
- If in doubt call for medical advice.
- If the child has difficulty breathing or shows signs of a lack of oxygen, **dial 999 for an ambulance.**

Meningitis

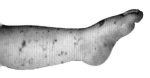

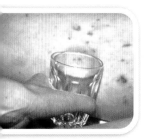

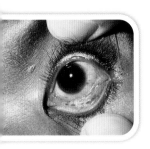

Meningitis is an inflammation of the linings surrounding the brain and spinal cord, which is caused by bacterial or viral infections.

One danger is that the signs and symptoms of meningitis can be easily mistaken for other common, less serious infections. A child with bacterial meningitis, however, often deteriorates rapidly.

Doctors should take the precaution of treating suspected cases *before* they get a definite diagnosis, because early treatment with hospital antibiotics is vital. A recent study showed that 50% of children with meningitis were initially sent home by their GP, so it is vital that you seek help again if the child gets worse – be persistent!

Possible signs and symptoms

'Red flag' early symptoms include:

- Cold hands and feet.
- Pain in the limbs or joints.
- Abnormal skin colour (pallor or mottling).

Other signs, which can occur later include:

- Fever *(high temperature)* and vomiting.
- Blotchy purple rash *(anywhere on the body)*. May start like pin pricks. It doesn't fade when it's squashed with a glass tumbler.
- Drowsiness or lowered levels of consciousness.
- Severe headache.
- Stiff neck *(can be rare)*.
- Dislike of bright lights *(can be rare)*.

With dark skin look for a pin prick rash in the skin under the eye.

The blotchy rash can be a late sign and it doesn't always occur, so don't wait for a rash to develop before you get help. Get advice early if you suspect meningitis could be developing.

More clues associated with babies:

- The soft spot on the baby's head may become tense or bulging.
- May refuse to feed, be irritable when picked up, or have a high pitched or moaning cry.
- May be fitting, or be floppy and lifeless, too sleepy to wake up.

Treatment

- Call the child's parents and the doctor. Explain why you are concerned, describe the symptoms carefully and ask for advice.
- If the doctor is not available go straight to the nearest casualty.
- If the rash is present, **dial 999 for an ambulance.**
- Be prepared to insist! If it's bacterial meningitis early treatment with hospital antibiotics is vital.

Pictures: Many thanks to the Meningitis Research Foundation. 24 hour free help-line: 080 8800 3344. www.meningitis.org

Diabetes

Diabetes is a condition suffered by a person who does not produce enough of a hormone called insulin.

Insulin works in your blood stream to 'burn off' the sugars that you eat. Some diabetic patients have such a lack of insulin, that they need to have insulin injections to keep their sugar levels down. This type of diabetic is called an 'insulin dependent' diabetic.

A child who is insulin dependent has to eat the right amount of sugar to match the insulin that's been injected. If the child doesn't eat enough sugar, the insulin injection will carry on burning off the small amount of sugar left in their blood stream, so the sugar levels may drop dangerously low.

Low blood sugar is dangerous because brain cells, unlike other cells in the body, can only use glucose *(sugar)* as their energy supply, so the brain is literally starved.

There are three common causes for a diabetic child's sugar levels to become low:

- *Missing a meal.*
- *Over exercising.*
- *Insulin overdose.*

Signs and symptoms of low blood sugar

- The condition usually starts and gets worse suddenly.
- Bizarre, uncharacteristic, uncooperative, possibly violent behaviour. Could be mistaken for 'drunkenness'.
- Confusion, memory loss.
- The child will deteriorate into unconsciousness if untreated.
- Pale, cold, sweaty skin.
- Shallow, rapid breathing and fast pulse.
- A diabetic patient may carry an insulin pen, glucose tablets, a warning card, or wear a medic-alert bracelet or necklace.

***DO NOT** attempt to give the child anything to eat or drink if they become unconscious.*

Treatment of low blood sugar

- Give the child a sugary drink *(isotonic sports drinks are best),* sugar lumps, glucose tablets, or other sweet foods.
- If the child responds to treatment quickly, give them more food or drink. Stay with them until they are fully alert and conscious.
- If the child doesn't respond to treatment within 10 minutes, or they are unmanageable, **dial 999 for an ambulance.**
- Consider if there is another cause for the child's symptoms.
- **If the child becomes unconscious,** maintain **Airway** and **Breathing** *(pages 10 to 13),* place them in the recovery position *(page 15)* and **dial 999 for an ambulance.**

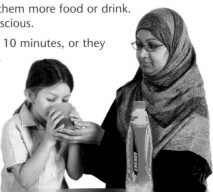

Other medical conditions

Fitting *(also called seizures or convulsions)* ?

There are many things that can cause a child to fit, such as epilepsy, a lack of oxygen to the brain, a head injury, or even the body temperature becoming too high.

If the fit is caused by a high temperature (which is common with young children), this is called a 'febrile convulsion'. See page 42 for more details.

The majority of fits follow a pattern of phases:

Aura If the child has had fits before, they may recognise that they are about to have one. The child may only get this 'warning' a few seconds before they fit.

Tonic Every muscle in the body becomes rigid. The child may let out a cry and will fall to the floor. The back may arch and the lips may go blue. This phase typically lasts less than 30 seconds.

Clonic The limbs of the body make sudden, violent jerking movements, the eyes may roll, the teeth may clench, saliva may drool from the mouth *(sometimes blood-stained as a result of biting the tongue)* and breathing could be loud like 'snoring'. The child may loose control of the bladder or bowel. This phase typically lasts less than 2 minutes.

Recovery The child stops fitting, and may go into a deep sleep or become very confused or agitated. The child should come around within a few minutes.

Treatment of fitting ✚

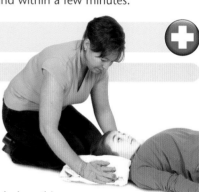

During the fit:

• Help the child to the floor to avoid injury.

• Move dangerous objects away from the child.

• Gently protect the head with a folded coat or your hands.

• Time the fit – make a note of the exact time and duration of fitting.

• Loosen any tight clothing around the neck to help breathing.

• **Dial 999 for an ambulance** if the fit lasts longer than **3 minutes**, they have a second fit, they have injured themselves, or this is the child's first ever fit.

After the fit:

• Check **Airway** and **Breathing** *(pages 10 to 13)*.

• Place the child in the recovery position *(page 15)*.

• Move bystanders away before they wake, to protect modesty.

• Dial 999 for an ambulance if you can't wake them up within **10 minutes**.

• Constantly monitor **Airway** and **Breathing**.

NEVER place anything in the child's mouth.

NEVER try to restrain the child.

NEVER move the child unnecessarily.

Body temperature

The body works best when its temperature is close to 37°C *(98.6°F)*. This temperature is maintained by an area in the centre of the brain called the *'hypothalamus'*.

If the body becomes too hot we produce sweat, which evaporates and cools the skin. Blood vessels near to the skin open up and the cooled blood is circulated around the body.

If the body becomes too cold we shiver, which creates heat by muscle movement. Blood vessels near to the skin close down *(pale skin),* keeping the blood close to the warmer core of the body. Tiny muscles pull tight to make the hairs on the skin stand up, trapping warm air *(goose pimples).*

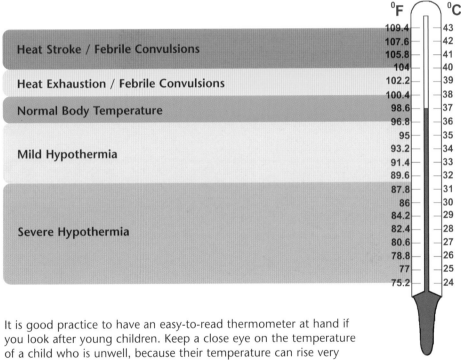

It is good practice to have an easy-to-read thermometer at hand if you look after young children. Keep a close eye on the temperature of a child who is unwell, because their temperature can rise very quickly *(see febrile convulsions, overleaf).*

Doctors often advise parents to give an unwell child mild painkillers such as paracetamol or ibuprofen. These drugs can help to prevent the temperature rising too high.

NOTE: *A child minder or carer should only give medication to a child if it is **prescribed by a doctor and they have written instructions from the parents**. It is very important to give the recommended dose only, and then inform the parents of the exact amount and time that the medication was given (page 46).*

Extremes of body temperature

Febrile convulsions

The area of the brain that regulates body temperature *(the hypothalamus)* is not fully developed until around 4 years old, so if a child develops an infection *(such as measles or tonsillitis),* this can lead to the core temperature of the body quickly rising.

The word febrile means 'related to fever' and indeed febrile convulsions are nearly always triggered by the child's temperature rising rapidly *(above 38°C).*

A febrile convulsion can be very frightening for the parents or carers of the child. During the first phase of the fit the child may appear to stop breathing and the lips may go blue. It goes without saying therefore, that if the parents are present, calm reassurance will be necessary *(see page 40 for more details about fitting).*

Febrile convulsions most commonly affect children between the ages of one and four *(they affect about 1 in 20),* but can affect children anywhere between six months and six years old.

The child may have been unwell over the past day or so and will be hot to touch.

Treatment of febrile convulsions

- Remove clothing and bedclothes. Provide fresh, cool air to cool the child down.
- Place the child on their side if possible to protect the **Airway**.
- Remove nearby objects and protect the child from injury whilst fitting. Pay particular attention to protecting the head.
- **Dial 999 for an ambulance.**
- If the child is still fitting – sponge them with tepid water to help the cooling process, but take care not to cool the child too much.
- Constantly monitor **Airway** and **Breathing** until the ambulance arrives *(pages 10 to 13).*

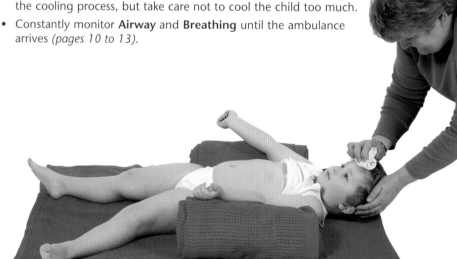

Heat exhaustion

Heat exhaustion is the body's reaction to loss of water and salt through excessive sweating. A typical episode would be a child that begins to feel poorly in the late afternoon or early evening, after exercising in very hot weather all day.

Heat exhaustion occurs when the core body temperature raises above 38°C. If the problem is not treated, it can quickly lead to heat stroke.

Possible signs and symptoms include:

- Confusion, dizziness.
- Pale, sweaty skin.
- Loss of appetite, nausea, vomiting, stomach cramps.
- The child may say that they 'feel cold', but they will be hot to touch.

Treatment of heat exhaustion

- Move the child to a cool shaded area. Remove excessive clothing and lay them down.
- Give the child a drink of water to re-hydrate them.
  If possible, add one level teaspoon of salt per litre of water.
- Obtain medical advice, even if the child recovers quickly.

Give the child a drink of water to re-hydrate them.

Heat stroke

Heat stroke is a very serious condition, and results in failure of the temperature control area of the brain. The sweating mechanism fails, the body is unable to cool down, and the body temperature can reach dangerously high levels *(over 40°C)*.

Possible signs and symptoms include:

- Severe confusion and restlessness. Lowered levels of consciousness, possibility of fitting.
- Flushed, hot, dry skin *(no sweating)*.
- Throbbing headache, dizziness, nausea, vomiting.

Treatment of heat stroke

- Move the child to a cool, shaded area.
- **Dial 999 for an ambulance.**
- Cool the child rapidly. Remove outer clothing and sponge with cold water, but take care not to over-cool the child.
- If the child fits, treat as a febrile convulsion *(opposite)*.

Extremes of body temperature

Hypothermia

NEVER give alcohol.

NEVER place direct sources of heat on or near the child.

NEVER try to warm young children or the elderly too quickly.

The onset of hypothermia occurs when the core body temperature falls below 35°C. The underlying cause of hypothermia is over exposure to cold temperatures, however other factors can increase the risk:

- Children under 4 years can be particularly at risk, as the temperature control area of the brain is not yet fully developed.
- Wet clothing, or immersion in cold water, results in the body cooling much faster than it would in dry air.
- A child who is not clothed properly in windy conditions will have cold air continually in contact with the skin, resulting in faster cooling of the body.

Possible signs and symptoms include:

- Pale skin, cold to touch.
- Shivering at first, then muscle stiffness as the body cools further.
- Slowing down of the body's functions: including thought, speech, actions, pulse, and breathing.
- Lethargy, confusion, disorientation *(can be mistaken for drunkenness)*, eventually unconsciousness, then death.

Treatment of hypothermia

For a conscious child:

- If you can shelter the child, remove any wet clothing. Quickly replace with dry, warm garments and cover the head.
- Wrap the child in warm blankets and cover the head. If indoors, heat the room to a warm temperature *(25°C)*.
- A child outdoors should be insulated from the environment and ground. Use a survival bag and shelter if available. Share body heat if necessary.
- Give the child a warm drink.
- Seek medical advice. If the condition seems severe, **dial 999 for an ambulance.**

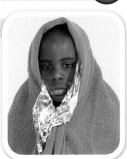

If the child becomes unconscious:

- Maintain **Airway** and **Breathing** *(pages 10 to 13)*.
- Very gently, place the child in the recovery position *(page 15)*. Place blankets or other insulating materials under and around the child, and cover the head. Do not move the child unnecessarily.
- **Dial 999 for an ambulance,** and constantly monitor breathing.

Dealing with an unwell child

It is important to contact parents as soon as possible if a child becomes injured or unwell. A frightened child will need comfort from a parent, and may not understand why they are not there when they need them so much.

Only a parent or legal guardian can give consent for medical treatment. Even if you have a 'medical consent form' already completed, medical staff will usually need direct permission from a parent if major treatment is required.

In the absence of a parent, a child may seek comfort from a person they trust, in which case, that person should stay with the child until the parent arrives. If the child has a favourite doll or cuddly toy, keep this with them if they need to go to casualty or the doctors.

Until a child is collected by parents:

- Take the child into a quieter environment away from other children if you can.

- Reassure the child. Try to take their mind off the situation.

- Keep an eye out for high temperatures. Remove excessive clothing and cool the child if necessary (pages 41 to 43).

- Having a vomit bowl on standby may prove useful!

- Use disposable towels for cleaning up body fluids (don't use the mop for the kitchen!). Protect yourself with disposable gloves and an apron if necessary.

- Clean body fluid spillages with effective cleaning agents.

- Wash your hands before and after dealing with the child to reduce the possible spread of infection.

Finding out what's wrong:

When trying to find out what's wrong with an injured or unwell child:

- Avoid asking 'leading' questions, such as 'does your tummy hurt?', because the inevitable answer from a poorly child would be 'Yes'!

- If you can, ask 'open' questions such as: 'What's the matter?', 'Do you hurt anywhere?', 'Can you point to it?', 'When did it start?'.

- If you check a child for injuries or pain, it's more comforting for the child if you start from the feet and work towards the head. Don't 'tower' over the child, sit or kneel as you talk to them.

- Use words that the child will understand: avoid adult terminology of body parts.

Giving medication

A child who has an infectious illness, or who feels poorly, should ideally be at home. Instances do occur, however, when another adult may be called upon to administer medication on behalf of a parent.

Before you agree to administer medication on behalf of a parent, it is strongly advisable that the following conditions are met:

- The child's parent or guardian should provide written, signed consent, giving clear instructions about dosage and timings.

- The medication should be prescribed by a doctor, and should be in its original packaging *(to prevent a parent from inappropriately administering medication, and you unwittingly helping them)*.

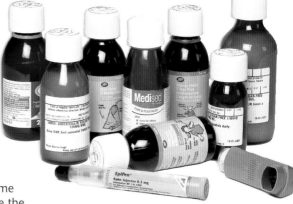

- The instructions from the parent should match the instructions on the pharmacy label or packaging.

- You should record the exact time and dosage each time you give the medication. Get the parent to read and sign this when they collect the child *(this is designed to prevent accidental overdose)*.

- For some medications, you may need training from a qualified medical professional *(if you were required to give an injection for example)*.

- You should store the medication in a safe place, out of sight and reach of children.

- Completed medication records should be stored safely in case they are required for insurance purposes at a later date.

A medication record book is available from the Pre-School Learning Alliance, or the National Child Minding Association:

www.pre-school.org.uk

www.ncma.org.uk

Accident recording

When caring for someone else's child, especially in the pre-school or childcare environment, it is important to make an accurate record of any accident, whilst the facts are fresh in everyone's head.

An accident record provides an accurate log of the circumstances surrounding an incident, so if an insurance claim should arise, perhaps at a later date, you are not having to rely on memory alone.

An injury which at first appears very minor can sometimes develop into a more serious condition, so it is important that the parents are informed of any accident involving the child, no matter how slight. Get the parent to sign the accident record when they collect the child.

Over a period of time, the accident record book may reveal a pattern of incidents that can be reviewed *(several injuries occurring whilst a child is playing a particular game for example)*, so action can be taken to prevent further accidents.

An accident record should be completed as soon as possible after the incident, and should contain the following information:

- Full name of the casualty.
- Name of the person who dealt with the accident.
- Date and time of the incident.
- The nature of what happened.
- The nature of the injury.
- The treatment given.
- What medical help was sought *(if any)*.
- Names of any witnesses.
- Layout of the incident area, including:
    - The layout of equipment in the area around the incident *(draw a sketch if possible)*.
    - The position of the child
    - The position of adults
- Further action required *(to prevent a re-occurrence)*.
- Parent's signature, to acknowledge that you have informed them about the accident.

An accident record book is available from the Pre-School Learning Alliance, or the National Child Minding Association:

www.pre-school.org.uk
www.ncma.org.uk

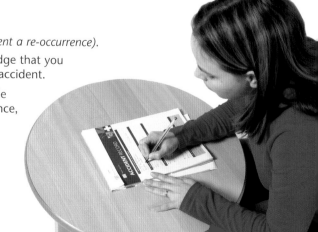

Useful advice

First aid kits

The following first aid kit list is based on a combination of advice from the Health and Safety Executive, the National Child Minding Association, the Pre-School Learning Alliance and colleagues from the Ambulance Service. The list is not mandatory, so equivalent or similar items can be used:

1 leaflet giving general guidance on first aid.

1 protective face shield for performing CPR.

20 individually wrapped sterile adhesive dressings of assorted size *(plasters)*. Only use 'hypo-allergenic' plasters for children, and blue coloured plasters for food handlers.

2 sterile eye pads.

4 triangular bandages, individually wrapped and preferably sterile.

6 medium wound dressings *(approx. 12cm x 12cm)*, individually wrapped and sterile. These have bandages attached.

2 large wound dressings *(approx. 18cm x 18cm)*, as above.

5 'low-adherent' dressings approx. 5cm x 5cm. These have a perforated plastic surface which reduces the likelihood of it sticking to the clotting blood. *(A popular brand is 'Melolin').*

5 'low-adherent' dressings, approx. 10cm x 10cm, as above.

1 roll of hypo-allergenic tape *(a popular brand is Micro-pore tape)*. Can be used to hold a dressing in place or fasten a bandage.

3 pairs of disposable gloves.

1 pair of scissors, with rounded ends.

10 'packs of 5' sterile gauze swabs, approx. 5cm x 5cm, for cleaning a wound *(don't use cotton wool because it can leave small particles in the wound)*.

1 finger bandage and applicator *(a popular brand is 'Tube-gauze')*.

If you have no clean tap water *(e.g. on a day trip)*:

1 litre of sterile water *(for cleaning wounds, washing eyes or immediate treatment of burns)*.

DO NOT *put sprays, antiseptic wipes, creams, lotions, tablets or medicines in a first aid kit intended for use on children.*

The quantity of items is suggested as the minimum you should have in your kit at any one time, so you may need to increase this for the number of children in your care, and replace items as soon as they are used.

Your first aid kit should be easily located by adults, and clearly identified by a white cross on a green background. The container should protect the contents from dust and damp.

The following questions are provided so you can test your knowledge of first aid. **Discuss with your first aid instructor which questions are best to revise.**

Write your answers on a separate sheet of paper. Answer the questions as best as you can from memory, then have a look in the book to mark yourself *(or improve your answers)*. The page numbers in *red italics* indicate where to look for the correct answer.

Attempt the questions again 3 months after your first aid course to see how much you have remembered!

1. **What are the priorities of treatment when dealing with a patient?** *Page 3*

2. **What modifications to the adult sequence of resuscitation can make it even more suitable for a child?** *Page 5*

3. **When performing chest compressions on a child or baby, how deep should you compress the chest?** *Page 5*

4. **If you were on your own, the nearest telephone was next door, and a child had stopped breathing, when should you leave them to dial 999 for an ambulance?** *Page 5*

5. **What is the ratio of chest compressions to rescue breaths when carrying out resuscitation?** *Page 8*

6. **If you were performing CPR on a child and they vomit, how can you tell this has happened? What should you do to clear the airway?** *Page 9*

7. **What are the 2 main dangers facing a child who is deeply unconscious and laid flat on her back?** *Page 15*

8. **A child in your care is playing with a very small toy. The next thing you see is him grasping his throat, unable to speak to you. What should you do?** *Page 16*

9. **A child has choked on some food and becomes unconscious. What should you do?** *Page 16*

10. **If a child had a life threatening allergic reaction, what signs and symptoms might you see?** *Page 19*

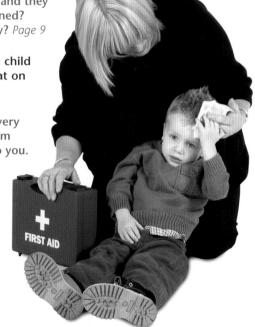

11. How would you treat a child having an asthma attack? *Page 20*

12. An infant starts to suffer from croup, what should you do? *Page 21*

13. What is the critical blood loss for a child weighing approx. 6 stones? *Page 22*

14. A child has lost a lot of blood. They look very pale and they are going dizzy when they stand up. What should you do? *Page 22*

15. A child has cut their forehead after falling outside and it's bleeding badly. There are no embedded objects in the wound. What should you do? *Page 23*

16. If a child gets a finger amputated, what should you do with the finger? *Page 24*

17. What should you do if a piece of glass is embedded in a wound? *Page 25*

18. How should you clean a graze? *Page 26*

19. Your next door neighbour's dog has just bitten their child. What first aid measures should they take? *Page 27*

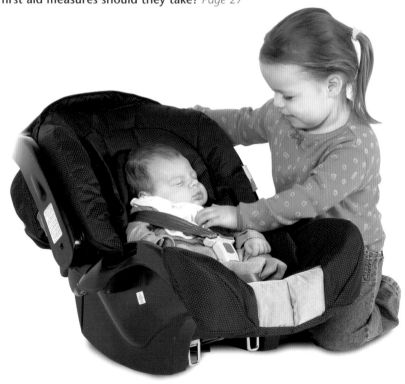

Test your knowledge

20. A child in your care has been stung by a bee. What should you do? *Page 27*

21. How should you treat a nose bleed? *Page 27*

22. A child has swallowed 30 of his mum's anti-depressant tablets. What should you do? *Page 29*

23. The following week, he drinks some bleach! What should you do now? *Page 28*

24. A very hot cup of tea gets spilt on a baby in a café. What should you do? *Page 30*

25. A child climbs into a high voltage electricity sub-station to retrieve a football. There is a loud bang and a flash of light. The child appears unconscious. What should you do? *Page 31*

26. A child is climbing in a tree in next door's garden. She falls and breaks her ankle. The bone has come through the skin. What is the best action to take? *Page 32*

27. What is the only way to tell the difference between a minor fracture and a sprain? *Page 33*

28. What is the best course of action if you think a child has sprained their wrist? *Page 33*

29. Which condition is worse, 'concussion' or 'compression'? *Page 34*

30. What is the main difference between the signs of 'concussion' and the signs of 'compression'? *Page 34*

31. What should you do if a child is knocked out because of a blow to the head? *Page 35*

32. A child is knocked down. He is breathing effectively, but he is unconscious. What should you do? *Page 36*

33. A child in your care suffers from sickle cell disease. What are the common triggers of a sickle cell crisis? *Page 37*

34. A baby in your care seems very poorly. Her condition seems to be getting worse by the hour. She doesn't like it when you pick her up and she is refusing to feed. What condition should you be aware of? What other signs should you keep an eye out for? What should you do? *Page 38*

35. A child in your care is an insulin dependent diabetic. He starts to act very strangely and becomes pale. What is probably wrong? What should you do? *Page 39*

36. A child has an epileptic fit. They are a known epileptic patient. What should you do during the fit? If the fitting continues, after how long should you dial 999 for an ambulance? *Page 40*

37. What temperature is 'normal' body temperature? *Page 41*

38. A 2-year-old starts fitting unexpectedly. They have been poorly all day and they feel very hot to touch. What should you do? *Page 42*

39. A child has been on a day out, walking in very hot weather. In the early evening he refuses to eat because he feels sick. He climbs into bed, shivering and looking pale. What is possibly wrong? What should you do? *Page 43*

40. A child is brought to you by a neglectful parent. The weather is freezing cold, it's raining, and she is not clothed properly. She is slurring her speech and very cold to touch. What should you do? *Page 44*

41. When questioning a child to find out what's wrong, it is important to avoid 'leading' questions. Give an example of a leading question. *Page 45*

42. What conditions should be met before you agree to administer medication on behalf of a parent? *Page 46*

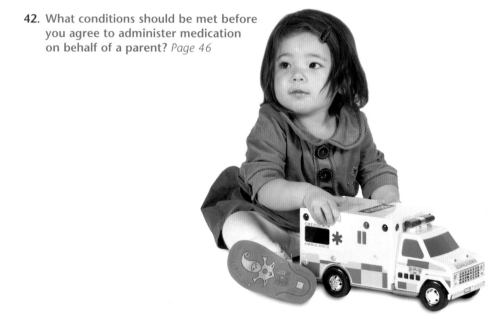